KETOGENIC DIET FOR BEGINNERS

SIMPLE 14-DAY KETO DIET PLAN WITH EASY RECIPES TO GET WEIGHTLOSS FAST AND EFFORTLESSLY MAXIMIZE PERFORMANCE

LOGAN WOLF

COPYRIGHT NOTICE

DISCLAIMER

Disclaimer Notice:

Please note the information contained within this document is for educational purposes only.

Every attempt has been made to provide accurate, up to date and reliable complete information no warranties of any kind are expressed or implied. Readers acknowledge that the author is not engaging in rendering legal, financial or professional advice.

By reading any document, the reader agrees that under no circumstances are we responsible for any losses, direct or indirect, which are incurred as a result of use of the information contained within this document, including – but not limited to errors, omissions, or inaccuracies.

TABLE OF CONTENTS

CHAPTER 1

INTRODUCTION

FITNESS AND DIETING are all the rage nowadays. As more people gradually abandon McDonald's in favor of Whole Foods and watching television on the couch for hitting the gym, the healthy lifestyle is becoming much trendier as time goes by. People are starting to realize the ill effects of junk food and lack of exercise. They are no longer taking their health for granted as they know that living a healthy life is part of living a quality life.

The thing is that most people dread the thought of having to go on a diet. Nobody wants to substitute the foods they love to eat for salads and yogurt all the time. Counting calories seems like a horrible way to lose weight.

But what if there was another option? What if there is a diet where you can eat plenty of high-fat foods and still lose weight? What if there was a diet that will never make you feel hungry? Lucky for you, there is. Welcome to the ketogenic diet.

CHAPTER 2

WHAT IS A KETOGENIC DIET?

THE KETOGENIC DIET, or keto diet for short, can be traced back all the way to 1921 when Dr. Rawle Geyelin found that ketosis was effective in treating epilepsy in children. In 1930, Dr. Clifford Barborka from the Mayo Clinic in Rochester, Minnesota studied 100 epilepsy patients in ketosis and found that 56% had a response rate of under 50% and 12% were completely free of seizures.

While the diet has historically been used to treat epilepsy patients, keto diets have gained mainstream popularity thanks to its unique approach that allows people to lose weight. The keto diet is a high-fat and low-carb diet that is somewhat similar to the Atkins diet.

The way the diet works is by ensuring that the dieter goes into a state of ketosis – a metabolic process where the body runs out of carbs to burn for energy, so it starts burning fat. This leads to a build-up of acids called ketones within the body.

Filling up your body with ketones is not only extremely effective at burning fat, but also provides tons of energy for your brain. Keto diets are also great at reducing blood sugar and insulin levels.

The fat burning helps stave off type 2 diabetes, pre-diabetes, metabolic syndrome, and a host of other nasty ailments. In fact, those on a keto diet can often reduce the amount of diabetes medication they need to take if not abandoning it altogether. One study published in *PubMed Central* found that 95.2% of those on the keto diet were able to take less or completely stop using their diabetic medication compared to only 62% of those on a higher carb diet. Another study found that one-third of type 2 diabetes patients on a keto diet were able to cease taking medications altogether.

Other studies have found that the keto diet can help reduce risk of brain injuries, cancer, tumors, acne, Alzheimer's disease, heart disease, Parkinson's disease, and more. Note that this research isn't completely conclusive and that more research should be conducted before we can get a full understanding of the diet's effects.

One major difference between keto diets and normal diets is that you won't need to count calories. While tracking what you eat is always a helpful thing to do, keto diets are flexible enough that you can still lose weight without downsizing your portions.

Keto diets also provide dieters with a lot of fat and protein, meaning that you will never go hungry and you won't be lacking the necessary protein your body needs. The increased protein take is also something that you won't often get from low-fat diets that restrict portion sizes.

How to Tell If You're in Ketosis

The optimal range of ketones in your body is between 0.5 and 3 mMol. That being said, having a high level of ketones doesn't necessarily mean you're in ketosis, but there are many signs that you might be.

The two most common signs of ketosis are smelly breath and

urine. Keto breath, as it is dubbed, it made because your body creates acetones when burning fatty acids. It gets rid of acetones through breath and urine, often leaving both with a "fruity" or slightly rotten smell. Keto breath is also accompanied by a slightly metallic taste in the mouth. You can use urine strips like Ketostix or breath takers to measure the ketone levels. Note that urine strips aren't always accurate since dehydration may result in a false positive and drinking too much can result in a false negative.

You will also lose a lot of water weight as your body flushes out the water stored in your muscles. This will often lead you to being dehydrated, so make sure to drink lots of water.

A glucometer can measure your blood sugar levels and tell if you're in ketosis. If your glucose levels are under 80mg/dl and you aren't hypoglycemic, then congratulate yourself as your body is using ketones for energy.

When your body finally adapts to ketosis, you will have high energy, better sleep, healthy blood sugar levels, no sugar cravings, a reduced appetite, less inflammation, less bloating, and less fatigue.

The keto diet clearly holds amazing potential as a way to become healthy without needing to starve yourself. Next, we will explore what happens when you finally start this diet.

CHAPTER 3

KETO FLU

IT'S VERY common for newcomers to the diet to experience what is known as keto flu. This is a host of flu-like symptoms caused from the fact that your body is no longer receiving the carbohydrates that it is used to getting.

Your body needs some time to adjust to its new diet. Keto flus usually last only one week, but in rare cases can stretch out to several weeks. It's different for everyone, but symptoms should disappear by or during your second week.

Common symptoms include dizziness, nausea, irritability, stomach pain, sugar cravings, fatigue, muscle cramping, and insomnia.

How to Fight Keto Flu

If you are experiencing keto flu symptoms, worry not. You can curb symptoms by making a few easy changes.

First, try eating more fats or calories. Your body needs energy and the lack of carbohydrates often means that you need to fill your body with healthy fats like olive oil coconut oil, tallow, or ghee. Adding more calories will also help give your body the energy it needs and you can refer to the food guide and the recipe list later on in this book.

Consuming more salts might be beneficial as well. Lower carbohydrates mean a lower insulin level which results in your body not holding onto as much sodium as it used to. Don't be afraid to add a little more salt since, if you are cutting out junk foods from your diet, you should already be consuming less salt than normal.

You will also want to keep well hydrated. Drinking water will help with headaches and nausea. You can also mix in sugarless electrolyte supplements to relieve symptoms like dizziness, muscle cramping, and fatigue. Drinks like Gatorade are high in electrolytes, but also contain a lot of sugar so you will want to avoid them. Instead, you can make your own keto-friendly elec-trolyte drink simply by mixing 1 tsp of mineral sea salt and lemon or lime juice with your water. You should especially take elec-trolytes if you regularly exercise while on the keto diet.

Another useful remedy is bone broth. It is incredibly healthy and provides water, fat, calories, and salt. You can make bone broth in your slow cooker by adding bones of your favorite meat, water, two tablespoons of apple cider vinegar for each gallon of water, and letting it sit for 10 hours. (Note: The vinegar helps draw the nutrients out of the bones.) When it's done cooking, simply strain it, package it, and refrigerate it. Your broth will prob-ably thicken in the fridge, so just heat it to liquefy it again. You can reuse the bones to make future servings of broth.

Note that when the broth cools, the fat will congeal and float to the top of the broth. You can eat the fat, but if it's too much for you, you can always scoop it out.

You could also take supplements to help with your keto flu. Exogenous ketone supplements such as Keto // OS or Perfect

Keto help raise ketone levels in your body, increase energy, and stave off fatigue.

If it's too hard for your body to recover from the carbohydrate withdrawal, you can simply slowly reduce your intake until your body becomes used to it. This just means that eating less and less carbohydrates every day until you reach the ideal level. Easing your body into fewer carbohydrates might be easier than just cutting it off all at once.

CHAPTER 4

FOOD AND SUPPLEMENTS

AS WITH ALL DIETS, a keto diet has a strict list of what you can and cannot eat. You might already be wincing at the thought of not being able to eat your favorite foods, but fear not. You have a lot of great choices when it comes to keto-friendly food. Just know that you want to avoid sugars and carbohydrates. In fact, you should aim for taking about 20-50 grams of carbohydrates a day, but it varies per person. Some sources will say that you should aim for 15 grams or less.

The below foods are all great and healthy options for ensuring that you get enough fat, protein, and oils. Try to opt for organic and grass-fed sources when possible.

Foods to eat:

- Meat: chicken, beef, eggs, lamb, steak, eggs, etc.
- Nuts and seeds: walnuts, peanuts, sunflower seeds, etc.
- Above ground vegetables and leafy greens: cauliflower, kale, cucumber, asparagus, etc.

- Berries: blackberries, raspberries, etc.
- High-fat dairy: hard cheese, full-fat yogurt, sour cream, cream cheese, heavy cream, etc.
- Sauces and condiments: yellow mustard, ketchup, horseradish, Worcestershire sauce, etc.
- Herbs and spices: rosemary, basil, thyme, cinnamon, nutmeg, cilantro, etc.
- Oils: olive oil, coconut oil, avocado oil, macadamia oil, etc.
- Sweeteners: monk fruit, stevia, saccharin, xylitol, etc.
- Beverages: water, broth, coffee, tea, coconut milk, almond milk, etc.

On the other hand, there are plenty of foods you want to avoid as well. Your carbohydrates should be limited as you'll get most of them from vegetables, nuts, and dairy. You also want to avoid most fruit due to their high sugar content, though avocados, berries, and star fruit can be eaten in moderation.

Foods to avoid:

- Fruit: apples, oranges, bananas, etc.
- Sugar: maple syrup, candy, honey, etc.
- Grains: bread, rice, pasta, cereal, etc.
- Below ground vegetables and tubers: potatoes, yams, carrots, radishes, etc.

Generally speaking, your diet should be about 70% fats, 25% protein, and 5% carbohydrates.

Supplements

You might want to boost your diet by taking supplements. Taking the right supplements can give you the essential vitamins and nutrients that you need to be fit and healthy. Supplements are obviously not completely necessary, but they can help accelerate your results by assisting with weight loss and increasing your energy levels. Supplements are especially useful for those going through keto flu. Note that supplements are meant to be taken in addition to a keto diet and are not a substitute for the actual diet.

Supplements to take:

- Keto // OS: This supplement provides you with exogenous ketones that will help your body fat right away even if you're not in ketosis. It's great for when you've taken too many carbohydrates, when you need to get your body back into ketosis, and when you need to relieve keto flu symptoms.
- Fish oil: Fish oil has two main benefits. First, it provides the body with much-needed omega-3s. Second, it's anti-inflammation properties can help combat some of the side effects of consuming too many fatty foods. Such foods are rich in omega-6s which are good for the body in small doses, but an excessive amount can lead to inflammation. Taking fish oil helps reduce inflammation and provides a healthy ratio of omega-3s and omega-6s.
- Perfect Keto: This product is almost identical to Keto // OS in that it helps provide exogenous ketones and fights symptoms of keto flu. The major differences between the two are prices and flavors.
- MCT oil: MCT stands for medium chain triglycerides, a fat molecule found in coconut oil, palm oil, and various dairy products. It's helpful for

reaching your daily fat intake and providing your body with the long-lasting energy it needs.

- Creatine: This amino acid is great if you're bodybuilding as it helps muscle contractions.
- L-Glutamine: This is another amino acid great for those with active lifestyles since working out sometimes reduces the amount of glutamine in the body. Additionally, cutting back on carbohydrates sometimes means you aren't getting the antioxidants you would otherwise be getting from fruits and vegetables. This is where L-glutamine comes in. Its antioxidant properties will not only keep you healthy, but will also increase your immunity, protect your muscles, and reduce recovery time after workouts.

CHAPTER 5

EXERCISE

MANY PEOPLE TRY to lose weight simply by eating less and working out more. This doesn't always work because the body needs a lot of energy especially when exercising. Cutting back on portions will just make you hungrier and fatigued and make it harder for you to resist the temptation of junk foods. Rather than eating less, you should strive to eat better.

Keto's high levels of protein make it great for ensuring that your muscles get what they need. When your body gets into ketosis, exercise can really help burn fat and give you a ton of energy.

The four main exercises you should know about are:

- Aerobic exercises, more commonly known as cardio, are any workouts that last over three minutes. They are low intensity and good for burning fat.
- Anaerobic exercises are exercises that require short bursts of energy such as high-intensity interval training and weight lifting. These types of workouts generally need carbs.
- Flexibility exercises are ones that require stretching your muscles and increasing your muscle's range of

motion. Yoga is probably the most well-known form of this.

- Stability exercises are ones that focus on balancing and training your core.

Remember that, when in ketosis, low-intensity exercises mostly use fat for energy while high-intensity exercises mostly use carbohydrates for energy. Athletes who perform high-intensity exercises are often on what is called the Targeted Keto Diet that involves eating their 20-50 grams of carbohydrates half an hour to an hour before their workout.

The longer one stays on a keto diet, the more adapted the body becomes to ketones. This means that the body becomes more and more efficient at burning fat and fueling itself by using ketones.

And you know what? It actually works. One study published by in *PubMed* found that athletes in a three-hour long run burned two to three times more fat if they were on a low-carb diet than if they were on a high-carb diet. Additionally, those on the low-carb diet used and replaced the same amount of muscle glycogen as the athletes in the high-carb group.

Note that the fuel and recovery provided by carbohydrates during high-intensity workouts is often unmatched by that of the keto diet. If you want to do low-intensity workouts and lose weight, keto is your answer. If you want to build a lot of muscle and compete in marathons and other contests, you might need to add some carbohydrates.

CHAPTER 6

SLEEP

GETTING enough sleep can be quite difficult when first starting a keto diet. The lack of carbohydrates that your body is so used to taking can cause insomnia and lead to many restless nights. Luckily, keto flu generally lasts about a week or so.

One reason that keto diets make it harder for you to sleep is because carbohydrates help the body produce L-tryptophan, which releases serotonin, which helps you sleep better. If you are having trouble sleeping, you may consider taking L-tryptophan supplements. Another solution is to eat a snack with protein and some carbohydrates before bedtime to increase insulin and serotonin levels.

Many people report needing less sleep while on a keto diet. While they would normally need eight to nine hours of sleep, they have gone down to a mere five or six hours, and still feel completely refreshed afterward.

CHAPTER 7

YOUR 14-DAY DIET PLAN

YOUR FIRST TWO weeks of keto will be the hardest, but they will likely be the most rewarding since they will set the foundation for your future diet. It will also be the time when you first experience keto flu, which can be off-putting for someone who is still new to the diet.

This guide is just a rough estimate of what you should be doing during your first two weeks. You don't have to follow it step-by-step, but it's good to have a handful of recipes that you like to fall back on. These are just a handful of recipes. You can find plenty more online.

Day 1

Breakfast: Bacon and Eggs

Ingredients:
2 eggs
2 slices of bacon
1 pinch of salt and pepper

Servings: 1

Steps:
Start off your keto diet with something you know
     and love! Fry your bacon in a pan until it's
     nice and crispy.
Fry the eggs in whichever style you choose.
Add salt and pepper and serve.

Lunch: Breadless Grilled Cheese

Ingredients:
2 eggs
1 tablespoons of almond flour
1 ½ tablespoons of psyllium husk powder
½ teaspoon of baking powder
3 tablespoons of butter
2 oz. cheddar cheese

Servings: 1

Steps:
Put 2 tablespoons of butter in a room temperature
     mug. When it turns soft, add the psyllium
     husk, baking powder, and almond flour.
Mix the ingredients together so that it makes a
     thick dough.
Crack the eggs, add to the mug, and keep mixing
     for a minute until it gets thicker.
Pour the dough mixture into a square container.
     Try and make it as even as possible.
Microwave it for 90-100 seconds.

Flip the container over so that the dough comes
out. It should now be solid and bread-like.

Cut it up into squares and put cheese between the
slices.

Put the remaining butter on a frying pan over
medium heat. Add the sandwiches and cook
until cheese is melted and "bread" is crisp and
then serve.

Dinner: Streak with Gremolata

Ingredients:

Streak:
2 small grass-fed ribeye steaks
1 pinch of salt and black pepper
1 tablespoon of butter

Gremolata:
2 cloves of mashed garlic
2 teaspoons of grated lemon zest
3 tablespoons of butter
4 tablespoons of chopped parsley

Servings: 2

Steps:
Let steak sit at room temperature for 10-15
minutes. Use a paper towel to clean off excess
blood.

Add salt, pepper, and melted butter.

Make the Gremolata by mixing melted butter,
parsley, lemon zest, and a tiny bit of salt.

Fry the steak in a pan over high heat for 2-4 minutes on each side until browned. Time may vary depending on how large your steak is and how well-cooked you want it to be.

Take the steak off and let it rest for 5-7 minutes. We recommend putting it in either a kitchen towel or parchment paper to keep it juicy.

When ready, serve with Gremolata.

Day 2

Breakfast: Coconut Porridge

Ingredients:
1 egg
1 tablespoon of coconut flour
4 tablespoons of coconut cream
1 pinch of ground psyllium husk powder
1 pinch of salt
1 oz. butter

Servings: 1

Steps:
Mix all your ingredients together in a non-stick saucepan on low heat. Keep stirring until you reach your ideal texture.
Eat it with coconut milk or cream and add toppings of your choice.

Lunch: Fat Head Pepperoni Pizza

Ingredients:

Pizza base:
1 ½ cups of grated mozzarella cheese
2 tablespoons of cream cheese
1 egg
½ teaspoon of salt
¾ cup + 1 tablespoon of almond flour
Extra virgin olive oil

Topping:
¼ cup of sugarless Marinara sauce
½ cup of grated mozzarella cheese
1/3 cup of grated parmesan cheese
3 oz. pepperoni
Basil
2 sliced jalapeno peppers (optional)

Servings: 4

Steps:
Preheat the oven to 425°F.
You'll make the crust by putting the mozzarella
    cheese and cream cheese into a bowl and
    microwaving on high for a minute. Then,
    use a spatula to mix the ingredients,
    microwave for another 30 seconds, and
    mix again.
Add egg, salt, almond flour, and mix.
Put the dough on a heatproof baking mat and
    flatten. You can put olive oil on your hands so
    keep it from sticking.
Bake the dough for 12-15 minutes.
Take out the dough and spread the marinara sauce
    on top. Add the cheese and pepperoni on top.

Add jalapeno peppers if you want. Put it back
  in the oven for 5 minutes.
Remove it from the oven and put basil on top.

Dinner: Spicy Cauliflower Soup

Ingredients:
1 large cauliflower
1 medium turnip
1 small white onion
1 medium Spanish chorizo sausage
2 cups of chicken stock
3 tablespoons of butter
½ teaspoon of salt
1 medium spring onion

Servings: 6

Steps:
Wash the cauliflower and cut it into florets.
Use the butter to grease a Dutch oven or a large
  soup pot. Add the chopped onion and cook over
  medium-high heat until lightly browned. Add
  the cauliflower and cook and stir for 5 minutes.
  Add the chicken, put on the lid, and cook for 10
  minutes before removing the heat.
Chop up the sausage. Peel and chop the turnip. Put
  them on a greased skillet and cook on medium-
  high heat for 8-10 minutes until the sausage is
  crispy and turnip is tender.
Put half of the sausage/turnip mix into the soup
  and use a hand blender to blend until the soup
  is creamy. Add salt and pepper.

Pour the soup into a bowl and add the rest of the
sausage/turnip mix. Add some chopped spring
onion and/or chives and then serve.

Day 3

Breakfast: Egg Muffins

Ingredients:
5 egg whites
2 whole eggs
3 lean breakfast turkey sausages
½ cup of skim milk
¼ cup of chopped spinach
¼ cup of shredded Cheddar cheese
1 pinch of salt and pepper

Servings: 6

Steps:
Preheat oven to 350°F.
Cook the sausage in a skillet over medium-high
heat until browned. Then remove them, cut
them into ½-inch pieces, and set aside.
Whisk egg whites and eggs in a large mixing bowl.
Add milk, salt, and pepper and keep whisking.
Then stir in the spinach.
Use cooking spray to grease up 6 cups in a muffin
tin or line those cups with paper liners. Pour
the egg mixture into those cups and then add
sausage and cheese.
Bake for 20 minutes or until solid. Let sit for 5
minutes to cool and serve.

Lunch: Low-Carb Vietnamese Pho

Ingredients:
8 cups of beef broth
1 medium white onion
1 4" piece of peeled ginger root
2 crushed garlic cloves
1 tablespoon of coconut aminos
1 tablespoon of fish sauce
2 packages of Shirataki noodles
1 pound of thinly sliced beef
Any additional toppings you desire

Servings: 4

Steps:
Freeze beef for 20 minutes to make it easy to slice.
Use a broiler to char the onion and ginger for 5-7 minutes until they turn black. Throw them in a soup pot with the garlic, coconut aminos, and fish sauce.
Pour the broth into the bowl.
Put the pot over a medium high heat until it boils. Then, reduce the heat to a simmer and cook for half an hour. Raise the heat again before you put the broth in the pot.
Prepare toppings and noodles.
Ladle the noodles and beef into bowls. Add any toppings you desire.

Lunch: Salad in a Jar

Ingredients:

4 oz. chicken 1 oz. leafy greens
1 oz. cherry tomatoes
1 oz. red bell peppers
1 oz. cucumber
½ scallion
4 tablespoons of mayonnaise or olive oil

Servings: 1

Steps:
Put your leafy greens on the bottom of the jar.
Chop your vegetables and add them in layers.
Top with chicken and add mayonnaise.
Serve. Feel free to mix up the vegetables, protein,
       and toppings to whichever you prefer.

Dinner: Bacon-Wrapped Cheese Burgers

Ingredients:

Filling:
2 tablespoons of butter
1 medium sliced white onion
2 ½ cups of sliced bell peppers
2 cups of sliced white mushrooms

Burgers:
1 kilogram of ground beef
10 slices of bacon
1 ¼ cups of shredded cheddar cheese
5 teaspoons of Sriracha
5 teaspoons of Dijon mustard
1 pinch of salt and pepper

Servings: 5

Steps:

Preheat the oven to 300°F.

Use the butter to grease a large frying pan. Cook
the sliced onions over medium-high heat for 5
minutes or until lightly browned.

Put in the sliced bell peppers and cook for another
5 minutes.

Put in sliced mushrooms and cook for another 3-5
minutes. Then take off the heat.

Divide the beef into five patties. Press the bottom of
a glass into the center of each patty to create a
pocket and fold the meat around the bottom of
the glass to make a bowl shape.

Wrap 2 slices of bacon around each "meat bowl"
and remove the glass by slowly twisting up.

Use the mixture you made earlier to fill up the "bowls"
in each patty. Then add Sriracha and Dijon
mustard to each patty. Top each off with cheese.

Place the patties on a baking sheet and bake them
for 45-60 minutes. Then remove them, let them
sit for 5 minutes, and serve.

Day 4

Breakfast: Scrambled Eggs with Halloumi Cheese

Ingredients:

4 eggs

4 oz. diced bacon
3 oz. diced halloumi cheese
8 tablespoons of chopped parsley
8 tablespoons of pitted olives
2 tablespoons of olive oil
2 scallions
1 pinch of salt and pepper

Servings: 2

Steps:
Heat up the olive oil in a frying pan on medium
     high heat. Fry the cheese, bacon, and scallions
     until they were decently brown.
Whisk the eggs and parsley in a bowl. Add salt and
     pepper.
Pour the mixture into the frying pan. Turn down
     the heat a little bit, add olives, and stir for a few
     minutes. Then you are ready to serve.

Lunch: Prosciutto Wrapped Mozzarella

Ingredients:
6 slices of prosciutto
18 leaves of fresh basil
1 container of Ciliegine mozzarella
1 pinch of salt and pepper

Servings: 6

Steps:
Cut the prosciutto into 1-inch sticks and roll

mozzarella into balls. Lay the strips next to
each other.

Put a basil leaf on the end of each strip with a
mozzarella ball on top.

Put some salt and pepper on top of the mozzarella.

Roll into the prosciutto and serve.

Dinner: Cauliflower Fritters

Servings: 1

Ingredients:
1 lb of raw cauliflower
1 teaspoon of salt
½ cup of almond flour
½ cup of grated cheese
½ teaspoon of baking powder
3 ounces of chopped onion
3 eggs
1 ½ teaspoons of lemon pepper

Steps:
Grate cauliflower and put it into a colander.
Sprinkle it with salt and mix using your hands.
Let it sit for 10 minutes.

Chop onions and put them in a medium bowl.
Squeeze the water out of the cauliflower and
put it into a medium bowl with the onions

Add cheese, almond flour, and baking powder.
Mix. Add eggs and mix more.

Place a skillet over medium heat and add a
tablespoon of oil. Scoop out the batter, ¼ cup at
a time, and place it onto the skillet. Flatten

with your spatula and cook for 3 minutes on
each side. Make sure not to flip until the
bottom is well-cooked.

Leave in the fridge. You can re-heat it in a dry
skillet at medium heat to make it crispy again.

Day 5

Breakfast: Keto Salmon and Cream Cheese Mug Muffin

Ingredients:

1 egg

2 tablespoons of cream or coconut milk

2 tablespoons of water

¼ cup of almond flour

¼ cup of flaxmeal

¼ teaspoon of baking soda

1 pinch of salt

60 grams of smoked salmon

2 tablespoons of chopped chives or spring onion

2 ounces of cream cheese

Servings: 2

Steps:

Add dry ingredients into a bowl and mix.

Add cream, water, and egg and mix.

Cut the salmon and chives and add them to the
bowl and mix.

Microwave for a minute and add cream cheese
on top.

Lunch: *Thai Fish and Coconut*

Ingredients:
1 ½ lbs of salmon
4 tablespoons of butter
2 tablespoons of red or green curry paste
13 ½ oz. coconut cream
1 oz. butter for greasing
8 tablespoons of chopped fresh cilantro
1 lb of cauliflower or broccoli
Salt and pepper

Servings: 4

Steps:
Preheat oven to 400°F and grease a baking dish.
Put the fish pieces in the baking dish. Fill as much
    as you can.
Add salt and pepper to the tops of the fish and then
    put a tablespoon of butter on top.
Mix the curry paste, cilantro, and coconut cream in
    a small bowl and then add the mixture to the
    top of the fish.
Bake for 20 minutes.
Boil your cauliflower or broccoli and serve with
    the fish.

Dinner: *Pork Chops with Blue Cheese Sauce*

Ingredients:
2 pork chops
1 ½ tablespoons of butter

3 ½ oz. blue cheese
3 ½ oz. green beans
2/3 cup of heavy whipping cream
1 pinch of salt and pepper

Servings: 2

Steps:
Crumble cheese into a small pot and put over
    medium heat until it melts, but not burns.
Add heavy cream, increase heat by a little, and let
    simmer.
Fry pork chops over medium heat. Add salt and
    pepper on one side for 2-3 minutes and then
    flip and cook again until the internal
    temperature is 145°-165°F. When done, take it
    out and cover it with foil for 2-3 minutes.
Pour the pan juices into the sauce and stir a little.
Trim and rinse the green beans. Fry the in butter
    and season with salt and pepper. Then serve.

Day 6

Breakfast: Scrambled eggs

Ingredients:
2 eggs
1 pinch of salt and pepper
1 oz. butter
1 splash of milk

Servings: 1

Steps:
Crack open some eggs in a bowl and whisk with a
    fork. Add milk to make it fluffier when cooked.
Melt butter onto a skillet or frying pan and put the
    whisked eggs on. Add some salt and pepper.
Cook until light and fluffy.

Lunch: Buttery Broccoli

Ingredients:
1 large bunch of cut broccoli
½ stick of butter cut into cubes
Salt and pepper

Servings: 6

Steps:
Put butter cubes into a mixing bowl and let it
    soften.
Cook broccoli in salted boiling water until tender.
    Then remove it.
Put the broccoli in the bowl with the butter cubes
    and toss the mixture so that the broccoli gets
    buttered.

Dinner: Sausages and Mash

Ingredients:

Sausages:
4 medium sausages
¾ small red onion
1 tablespoon of butter

Mash:

2/3 small cauliflower with stalk and leaves
    removed
½ medium peeled celeriac
1 heaped tablespoon of butter
1 pinch of salt and pepper

Servings: 2

Steps:

Put the sausages in a greaseproof lined baking tray.
    You may cut them lengthwise if you prefer.
Peel and slice onions and put them in the same
    tray. Drizzle them with some butter and toss.
Roast both in the oven for 30 minutes until cooked.
Create the mash by putting a pan of boiling water
    on the hob. Remove all stalks, leaves, and skin
    from cauliflower and celeriac and chop them
    before putting them into the boiling water. Boil
    for 15 minutes until soft.
Drain the water, dry off, and then put it into a food
    blender. Don't fully blend it or it will turn
    soupy. Just blend in small bursts until it's
    slightly thick.
Remove mash and serve with sausage.

Day 7

Breakfast: Healthy Pancakes with Cream Cheese Topping

Ingredients:

5 eggs
9 oz. cottage cheese
1 pinch salt
1 tablespoon ground psyllium husk powder
2 oz. butter

Topping:
8 oz. cream cheese
2 tablespoons of olive oil
2 tablespoons of green or red pesto

Servings: 4

Steps:
Mix the cream cheese, 1 tablespoon of olive oil, and
    pesto for the topping.
Put the eggs, salt, cottage cheese, and psyllium husk
    powder into a hand blender and mix until it
    becomes a batter. Let it sit for 10 minutes.
Heat up the butter on a frying pan and put drop
    some of the pancake batter onto the surface so
    that they form small circular shapes.
Fry the batter until they become solid pancakes.
    Serve with the cream cheese topping and
    sprinkle the rest of the olive oil on top.

Lunch: Shrimp and Sausage Skewers

Ingredients:
1 package of cooked sausage
1 ½ lbs of large raw, peeled, deveined shrimp
2 garlic cloves
½ teaspoon of salt

½ teaspoon of pepper
¼ cup of melted butter

Servings: 8

Steps:

Whisk chili pepper, garlic, butter, salt, and pepper together in a bowl.

Cut each sausage in 8 slices. Put one slice on each skewer with the cut part face down. Then add the shrimp so that it curls around the sausage. Repeat until skewer is full.

Brush each skewer with the mixture you made in step 1.

Grill each side about for about 2-3 minutes until shrimp is cooked.

Add salt and pepper.

Dinner: Keto Tuna Salad

Ingredients:
1 small head of lettuce
140 grams of tinned and drained tuna
2 hard-boiled eggs
2 tablespoons of mayonnaise
1 medium spring onion
1 tablespoon of fresh lemon juice
1 tablespoon of extra virgin olive oil
1 pinch of salt

Servings: 1

Steps:

Tear the lettuce leaves. Wash them and drain them
and spread them in a serving bowl.

Add the tuna.

Chop the hard-boiled eggs and add them to
the salad.

Mix the mayonnaise and lemon juice and add that
to the top of the salad. Then chop the spring
onion before adding that to the salad. Chives
work too.

Drizzle with olive oil and serve.

Day 8

Breakfast: Breakfast tapas

Ingredients:
Variety of cold cuts
Variety of cheese
Nuts
Cucumbers, pickled cucumbers, peppers, and
radishes
Avocado with mayonnaise and pepper
Basil

Serving size: 4

Steps:
Chop up the cold cuts, cheeses, and vegetables into
blocks or sticks.
Split open the avocado and cut it into wedges.
Mix with the mayonnaise.
Put the ingredients in avocado shells and serve.

Lunch: Cajun Chicken Tacos

Ingredients: 1 package of boneless skinned chicken
     thighs
½ medium red onion
½ juiced lime
2 garlic cloves
1 tablespoon of oregano
1 tablespoon of thyme
¼ teaspoon of cayenne pepper
½ teaspoon of paprika
2 tablespoons of butter
Coconut milk
2 heads of small lettuce
1 pinch of salt and pepper

Servings: 2

Steps:
Peel and chop the onion. Mash the garlic.
     Chop herbs.
Dice the chicken and mix with herbs, paprika,
     black pepper, garlic, and cayenne. Then add
     salt and lime juice.
Melt butter on a skillet over medium heat. Then
     add the herbed chicken and cook for about 10
     minutes.
Add cream and cook and stir for another 2-3
     minutes.
Wash and drain lettuce and then put the chicken
     on top.

Dinner: Pork and Halloumi Fat Stacks

Ingredients:

Burgers:
1 lb of ground free-range pork sausage
10 green chopped olives
1 egg yolk
1 tablespoon of Lemon Garlic seasoning

Toppings:
1 package of Halloumi cheese
1 avocado
½ cup of micro greens
1 cup of arugula
4 tablespoons of picked red onions

Steps:
Mix the burger ingredients in a bowl to make 4
    patties.
Grill each burger on both sides.
Serve them on arugula or wrapped in lettuce.
Grill the Halloumi cheese and add that to the top
    of the burgers along with the other toppings.

Day 9

Breakfast: Keto Breakfast Hash

Ingredients:
2 slices of bacon
1 egg
1 medium zucchini

1 clove of garlic or ½ of small white onion
1 tablespoon of coconut oil or ghee
1 tablespoon of chives of chopped parsley
¼ teaspoon of salt

Servings: 1

Steps:
Peel and chop the garlic or onion and slice
the bacon.
Put both in a frying pan over medium heat and stir
until lightly browned.
Dice zucchini into small pieces.
Add zucchini to the frying pan and cook 10-15
minutes. Then, take out your food and add the
parsley.
Add a fried egg on top and eat.

Lunch: Egg-Stuffed Avocado

Ingredients:
1 large avocado or 2 medium avocados
4 large eggs
¼ cup of mayonnaise
2 tablespoons of sour cream
1 teaspoon of Dijon muster
2 medium spring onions
1 pinch of salt
Ground black pepper

Servings: 2

Steps:

Fill a saucepan 3/4th of the way with water. Add a
   bit of salt. Boil the water. Carefully use a spoon
   to dip each egg in and out of the water. You
   will need about 10 minutes for them to become
   fully hard-boiled.
Take the eggs out when done and dice them. Slice
   the spring onion as well.
Add them to a bowl and mix with mayonnaise, sour
   cream, and Dijon mustard. Make sure to leave out
   some onion for garnish. Add some salt and pepper.
Scoop out the middle of the avocado and cut the
   part you took out into tiny pieces.
Place those avocado pieces into the bowl and mix.
Fill the avocado shell with the mixture and add a
   bit of spring onion on top.

Dinner: Low-Card Spaghetti Bolognese with Zucchini Noodles

Ingredients:
1 zucchini
1 chopped onion
2 crushed garlic cloves
500 grams of mince/ground beef
400 grams of canned chopped tomatoes
Italian herbs of your choice (rosemary, oregano,
   sage, basil, etc.)
1 pinch of salt and pepper

Servings: 5

Steps:

Create your "zoodles" by chopping off the ends of
   your zucchini and putting it through a
   spiralizer machine.

Fry onion and garlic in oil until soft, but not
   overcooked.

Add the beef and keep frying and stirring until all
   the beef is cooked.

Add the seasoning, tomatoes, and herbs.

Stir, simmer, and serve with zoodles and cheese
   on top.

Day 10

Breakfast: Low-Carb Frittata with Spinach

Ingredients:

8 eggs

1 cup of heavy whipping cream

5 oz. shredded cheese

5 oz. chorizo or diced bacon

2 tablespoons of butter

1 pinch of salt and pepper

Servings: 4

Steps:

Preheat the oven to 350°F.

Cook the bacon until it's crispy and add the
   spinach.

Whisk the eggs and cream and pour the mixture
   into a greased baking dish.

Add the bacon and spinach and bake for 25-30
minutes.

Lunch: Pork Schnitzel

Ingredients:
4 pieces of pork schnitzels
100 grams of almond meal or flour
1 tablespoon of dried rubbed sage
2 eggs
Oil for frying
1 pinch of salt and pepper

Servings: 1

Steps:
Beat the eggs with a fork in a small dipping bowl.
In a different bowl, add almonds, sage, salt, and
pepper.
Dip 1 pork schnitzel in the egg and let drain. Then
place it in the other mixing bowl and turn a
few times until it's covered.
Place each pork schnitzel in the frying pan. Cook at
a medium heat until both sides are golden
brown and serve.

Dinner: Steak with Mustard and Peppercorn Sauce

Ingredients:

Steaks:
2 small boneless steaks

1 tablespoon of butter
1 pinch of salt and pepper

Mustard and Peppercorn Sauce:
1 tablespoon of butter
1 tablespoon of peppercorns
1 tablespoon of Dijon mustard
½ teaspoon of onion powder
¼ cup of heavy whipping cream
¼ cup of bone broth
1 pinch of salt

Servings: 2

Steps:
Let steak sit at room temperature for 10-15 minutes. Use a paper towel to clean off excess blood.
Fry the steak in a pan over high heat for 2-4 minutes on each side until browned. Time may vary depending on how large your steak is and how well-cooked you want it to be.
When the steak is done cooking, lightly cover it with foil and let sit for about 10 minutes before serving.
Prepare the sauce by adding the leftover butter to the pan. Crush the peppercorns with a rolling pin and add them to the pan. Cook over medium-high heat for 2-3 minutes.
Add the other sauce ingredients and bring to a boil. Reduce the liquid by half and then cook for 3-5 minutes until creamy.
Serve the sauce with steaks.

Day 11

Breakfast: Breadless Breakfast Sandwich

Ingredients:
4 eggs
2 tablespoons of butter
1 oz. ham
2 oz. cheddar cheese
1 pinch salt and pepper
A few drops of Worcester sauce

Servings: 2

Steps:
Fry eggs over easy and add salt and pepper.
Use a fried egg for a bread substitute. Place your ham (or whichever meat you chose) on each egg and add the cheese. Place another fried egg on top of each stack to create your sandwich.
Add some sauce to the top and you're ready to eat.

Lunch: Turkey with Cream Cheese Sauce

Ingredients:
1 1/3 lbs of turkey breast
2 tablespoons of butter
2 cups of heavy whipping cream
7 oz. cream cheese
1/3 cup of small capers
1 tablespoon of soy sauce
1 pinch of salt and pepper

Servings: 4

Steps:
Preheat oven to 350°F.
Melt half the butter into an oven-proof frying pan
    over medium heat. Season with salt and pepper
    and sauté the turkey until golden brown.
Cook the turkey in the oven. When it's ready, take
    it out, put it on a plate, and cover in foil.
Poor the drippings into a small saucepan and add
    whipping cream and cream cheese. Stir, bring
    it to a light boil, and then lower the heat and
    simmer until it gets thick. Add salt and pepper.
Put the remaining butter in a frying pan over high
    heat. Sauté with capers until they become
    crispy and then serve with turkey.

Dinner: Oven Baked Keto Fried Chicken

Ingredients:
12 chicken drumsticks
4 cups of unsweetened almond milk
4 tablespoons of lemon juice
2 tablespoons of sea salt
2 teaspoons of ground black pepper
2 teaspoons of smoked paprika
2 teaspoons of dried oregano
1 teaspoon of onion powder
1 teaspoon of garlic power
1 ¼ cup of pork rinds
¼ cup of coconut flour
Olive oil

Servings: 6

Mix almond milk, lemon juice, salt, pepper, and
    oregano into a bowl.
Put the chicken pieces in a brine for anywhere from
    90 minutes to overnight.
When the brine is finished, add the other
    ingredients except for the cooking oil into a
    food processor and pulse until everything is
    combined into crumbs.
Preheat oven to 360°F.
Put the new crumbled coating into a tray. Dip the
    chicken pieces into the coating and roll until
    coated.
Put the chicken pieces onto a lined baking tray.
    Bake for about 45 minutes depending on how
    big the pieces are. Remove the tray halfway
    through the baking time to spray the pieces
    with olive oil and put the back in.

Day 12

Breakfast: Low-Carb Porridge

Ingredients:
1 tablespoon of whole flax seeds
1 tablespoon of chia seeds
1 tablespoon of sunflower seeds
1 cup of coconut milk or unsweetened almond
    milk
1 pinch of salt

Servings: 1

Steps:

Mix everything together in a small sauce span. Put
the heat on low and have the mix simmer until
it's at your ideal level of thickness.

Put whatever topping you want on it and eat it.

Lunch: Chili Covered Salmon with Spinach

Ingredients:

1 ½ lbs of salmon
1 tablespoon of chili paste
1 cup of mayonnaise
4 tablespoons of grated parmesan cheese
1 lb of spinach
1 oz. butter
1 pinch of salt and pepper

Servings: 4

Steps:

Preheat oven to 400°F.

Grease a baking dish with half of your butter. Slice
the salmon and add salt and pepper. Add it to
the dish face down.

Mix chili paste, cheese, and mayonnaise together
and spread the mixture onto the salmon pieces.

Bake for 15-20 minutes or until the salmon can be
flaked with a fork.

Sauté the spinach in the rest of the butter for about

2 minutes until wilted and add salt and
pepper.
Serve the spinach with salmon.

Dinner: Salmon and Avocado Omelet

Ingredients:
3 eggs
½ avocado
½ package of smoke salmon
2 tablespoons of cream cheese
2 tablespoons of chopped chives
1 medium spring onion
1 tablespoon of butter
1 pinch of salt and pepper

Servings: 1

Steps:
Crack eggs into a mixing bowl. Add salt and
pepper and beat the eggs.
Mix cream cheese and chives. Slice salmon and
peel and slice the avocado.
Grease a frying pan with butter and pour the eggs
in. Use the spatula to bring the eggs to the
center for the first 30 seconds and cook for 1-2
minutes.
Your eggs should form a nice shell. Bring it onto a
plate and put the cheese spread on top.
Add the salmon, avocado, and onions. Fold into a
wrap and serve.

Day 13

Breakfast: Crustless Mini Quiche

Ingredients:
6 eggs
6 slices of bacon
50 g shredded cheese
1 pinch of salt and pepper

Servings: 6

Steps:
Line the cups in a cupcake pan with bacon and make sure that the sides are completely covered.
Crack an egg in each cup.
Add cheese, salt, and pepper to each cup.
Bake at 350°F for 15 minutes.

Lunch: Breadless BLT

Ingredients:
4 slices of bacon
1 sliced tomato
2 romaine leaves
2 tablespoons of mayonnaise
1 pinch of salt and pepper

Servings: 1

Steps:

Put mayonnaise on the lettuce leaves. Then add
    salt and pepper.
Put two strips of bacon on each leaf. Then add
    tomatoes.
Put the two together to create your wrap.

Dinner: Chops in Red Pesto

Ingredients:
2 pork chops
1 tablespoon of butter
3 tablespoons of red pesto
4 tablespoons of mayonnaise

Servings: 2

Steps:
Rub the pork chops with 2 tablespoons of red
    pesto. Fry on a skillet over medium heat in
    butter for 8 minutes and then let simmer for 4
    minutes.
Mix the mayonnaise with the rest of the red pesto
    for pesto mayonnaise.

Day 14

Breakfast: Spinach and Feta Omelet

Ingredients:
3 eggs
1 clove of garlic
1 cup of sliced white mushrooms
3 cups of spinach

1/3 cup of crumbled feta cheese
2 tablespoons of butter
1 pinch of salt and pepper

Servings: 2

Steps:
Dice garlic and place into a pan after the pan has
    been greased with butter. Add salt and cook at
    medium-high heat for a minute.
Add sliced mushrooms and stir occasionally for 5
    minutes until lightly browned.
Add spinach and cook until wilted. Put your
    mixture into a bowl and dispose of any liquids.
Crack eggs into a separate bowl and add salt and
    pepper.
Pour the cracked eggs into the pan until the texture
    is soft and fluffy.
Add the filling to the new omelet shell and fold the
    omelet. Keep on the pan for a bit to keep it
    heated and then serve.

Lunch: Chicken Breast with Herb Butter

Ingredients:
4 chicken breasts
1 oz. butter
1 pinch of salt and pepper
8 oz. of spinach

Herb butter:
5 oz. butter
1 garlic clove

½ teaspoon of garlic power
1 teaspoon of lemon juice
½ teaspoon of salt
4 tablespoons of parsley

Servings: 4

Steps:
Mix all herb butter ingredients in a bowl and let
    it sit.
Add salt and pepper to the chicken. Fry it in butter
    at medium heat until cooked. Use a meat
    thermometer to make sure that the chicken is at
    165 degrees. You can lower the heat too to
    make sure the chicken doesn't end up too dry.
Put the chicken on top of leafy greens and add herb
    butter.

Dinner: Chicken and Spinach Pizza

Ingredients:

Pizza base:
1 ½ cups of grated mozzarella cheese
2 tablespoons of cream cheese
1 egg
½ teaspoon of salt
¾ cup + 1 tablespoon of almond flour
Extra virgin olive oil

Toppings:
1 boneless skinless chicken breast
½ tablespoon of olive oil

1 minced garlic clove
½ cup of heavy whipping cream
½ teaspoon of xantham gum
1 cup of chopped spinach
½ cup of shredded mozzarella
1 pinch of salt and pepper

Servings: 2

Steps:
Preheat the oven to 425°F.
You'll make the crust by putting the mozzarella
    cheese and cream cheese into a bowl and
    microwaving on high for a minute. Then, use a
    spatula to mix the ingredients, microwave for
    another 30 seconds, and mix again.
Add egg, salt, almond flour, and mix.
Put the dough on a heatproof baking mat and
    flatten. You can put olive oil on your hands so
    keep it from sticking.
Bake the dough for 12-15 minutes.
Sauté the chicken in a skillet over medium heat
    and then set aside.
Add garlic, xantham gum, and heavy whipping
    cream to the skillet and boil. Reduce to simmer
    when the sauce thickens.
Add spinach and cook until wilted.
Add the sauce to pizza dough and top with chicken
    and cheese.
Bake for 5 minutes and then serve.

CHAPTER 8

STAYING COMMITTED

STAYING COMMITTED to any diet is always hard work. It might be even harder on a keto diet when you realize that you can't eat the high-carb foods that you've been eating all your life. Having to be picky about every single meal you eat isn't an easy thing at all, but that doesn't mean it's not worth it.

Think of it this way: What are the things you really want in life? Unless you encounter some miracle, such as winning the lottery, you will never achieve your goals unless you go through a bit of struggling. Everything good in life comes through hard work and adversity. The harder you work now, the more you can reap the benefits in the future. Take this quote from blogger and author Mark Manson:

"Everybody wants to have great sex and an awesome relationship — but not everyone is willing to go through the tough conversations, the awkward silences, the hurt feelings and the emotional psychodrama to get there. And so they settle. They settle and wonder 'What if?' for years and years until the question morphs from 'What if?' into

'Was that it?' And when the lawyers go home and the alimony check is in the mail they say, 'What was that for?' if not for their lowered standards and expectations 20 years prior, then what for?

Because happiness requires struggle. The positive is the side effect of handling the negative. You can only avoid negative experiences for so long before they come roaring back to life.

What determines your success isn't 'What do you want to enjoy?' The question is, 'What pain do you want to sustain?' The quality of your life is not determined by the quality of your positive experiences but the quality of your negative experiences. And to get good at dealing with negative experiences is to get good at dealing with life."

How much do you want to get out of your current situation? Perhaps your life insurance is way too high. Maybe you don't like the way you look in your Facebook profile picture. You might be getting winded trying to walk up a set of stairs. Now think about what you might look like in the future. Slim, fit, and healthy. How much work are you willing to put in to get that?

You should also know that you're not the only one going through this. Listen to keto podcasts. Read blogs like *Keto Diet App*, *Peace Love and Low Carb*, *Ketogasm*, and *Wicked Stuffed*. Find others who are going through the same thing and learn as many tasty recipes you can. Go to subreddits like /r/keto and /r/ketorecipes where you can talk to others who have been where you are and are loving every second of their keto diet.

Lastly, get an app to keep track of your progress. MyFitnessPal is probably the easiest place to start so you can jot down how many carbs you eat per day and how close you are to reaching your goal. Keeping a food diary might sound tedious, but it allows you to look back at your progress and see how far you've gone and how much further you need to go.

CHAPTER 9

CONCLUSION

THIS BOOK IS JUST a jumpstart to getting your awesome keto diet off the ground. It's a handy way to find out how to best start your new lifestyle and how to keep it going, but it's always helpful to do your own research. Perhaps you won't like the 21 recipes provided here, and that's okay. There are hundreds of keto recipes floating around on the internet and all it takes it a few clicks to find the ones you do like.

This book might not provide you with everything you need to know for a lifelong diet, but it should get you started on something that can potentially change your life. You will be happier and healthier, but not hungrier. Know that sticking with your diet can lead to some fantastic results you wouldn't have been able to imagine otherwise.

Happy dieting and keep up the excellent work.

Made in the USA
Middletown, DE
15 January 2019